Natural Healthy Weight Loss with Sugar Defender

PROBLEM WITH BLADE SUGAR LEVEL, DIABETES, WEIGHT LOSS, LOOKING AND FEELING BETTER, SLIMMER BODY, HEALTHIER, MORE ENERGETIC,

HENRYK

Contents

Introduction ... 7

1. UNDERSTANDING BLOOD SUGAR AND WEIGHT LOSS ... 9
   1.1 The Science of Blood Sugar in Weight Management ... 9
   1.2 How Sugar Defender Helps Stabilize Blood Sugar ... 11
   1.3 Identifying Personal Blood Sugar Triggers ... 12
   1.4 The Impact of Unstable Blood Sugar on Your Health ... 13
   1.5 Natural Ingredients in Sugar Defender and Their Benefits ... 14
   1.6 Setting Realistic Goals for Blood Sugar Management ... 16

2. DIETARY APPROACHES TO SUPPORT BLOOD SUGAR BALANCE ... 19
   2.1 Crafting a Low-GI Meal Plan for Long-Term Health ... 19
   2.2 Deciphering Carbohydrates ... 21
   2.3 The Role of Fiber in Managing Blood Sugar Levels ... 22
   2.4 Optimal Protein Sources for Regulating Blood Sugar ... 24
   2.5 Essential Fats for Optimal Health and Weight Management ... 25
   2.6 Mastery of Food Labels: The Key to Unveiling Hidden Sugars ... 26

3. RECIPES AND MEAL PLANNING ... 29
   3.1 Energizing Breakfast Ideas ... 29
   3.2 Balanced Light Lunches ... 30
   3.3 Blood Sugar-Friendly Dinners ... 31
   3.4 Smart Snacking Strategies ... 32

3.5 Guilt-Free Desserts 33
3.6 Mastering Meal Preparation 34

4. LIFESTYLE MODIFICATIONS FOR BETTER BLOOD SUGAR 37
4.1 Regular Physical Activity 37
4.2 Sleep: The Essential Foundation of Blood Sugar Stability 39
4.3 Effective Stress Management for Optimal Blood Sugar Control 40
4.4 Lifestyle Choices 41
4.5 Evaluating Natural Supplements for Blood Sugar Management 42
4.6 Maintaining Motivation and Monitoring Progress 43

5. OVERCOMING CHALLENGES AND COMMON OBSTACLES 49
5.1 Overcoming Sugar Cravings 49
5.2 Navigating Dining Out 50
5.3 Navigating Social and Holiday Eating 52
5.4 Breaking Through Weight Loss Plateaus 53
5.5 Coping with Setbacks 54
5.6 Successfully overcoming the hurdles of sugar cravings. 55

6. SUCCESS STORIES AND MOTIVATIONAL INSIGHTS 59
6.1 From Pre-Diabetic to Empowered: John's Journey 59
6.2 Losing Weight and Gaining Energy: Lisa's Story 61
6.3 Managing Type 2 Diabetes 61
6.4 A Family's Journey to Better Health 62
6.5 Overcoming PCOS and Insulin Resistance: Anna's Tale 62
6.6 The Role of Community Support in Successful 63

7. ADVANCED STRATEGIES FOR BLOOD SUGAR MANAGEMENT — 65
7.1 Intermittent Fasting: Is It Right for You? — 65
7.2 The Keto Diet and Blood Sugar Control — 67
7.3 Advanced Carb Counting for Fine-Tuned Control — 68
7.4 Supplements and Herbs: A Deeper Dive — 71

8. MAINTAINING YOUR GAINS AND PREVENTING RELAPSE — 79
8.1 Setting Up a Long-Term Maintenance Plan — 79
8.2 Regular Check-Ups and When to Seek Professional Help — 81
8.3 Educating Friends and Family on Your Lifestyle Choices — 82
8.4 Adjusting Your Plan as You Age — 84
8.5 The Importance of Continuous Learning and Adaptation — 86
8.6 Celebrating Your Success and Planning for the Future — 87

Conclusion — 91
References — 95

Introduction

Every day, many individuals struggle with blood sugar imbalances, persistent sugar cravings, and weight management challenges. These battles extend beyond numbers, reflecting deeper quests for control, health, and vitality. My journey has been no different, propelling me to discover effective and sustainable solutions. Sugar Defender emerges as a beacon of hope for those navigating the complexities of diabetes and weight loss. This non-GMO supplement, formulated with natural ingredients, aims to stabilize blood sugar levels naturally. Its innovative approach positions it as a supplement and a pivotal component of a healthier lifestyle.

This book provides a comprehensive guide to natural weight loss, diabetes management, and overall health enhancement with Sugar Defender's support. Our holistic strategy encompasses diet, exercise, and mental well-being, offering a complete blueprint for your health transformation. The critical role of stable blood sugar levels in preventing diabetes, obesity, and cardiovascular diseases cannot be overstated. With millions worldwide affected by these conditions, there's a pressing need for effective interventions. Distinctively, this book integrates Sugar Defender into a wider lifestyle modification framework. It's not solely about changing your diet but transforming your life.

Through the lens of blood sugar science and real-life success stories, we aim to provide the knowledge and resources needed for a significant lifestyle change. This book is targeted at individuals dealing with sugar-related health issues, both newcomers to blood sugar management and those who have long faced such challenges. Our advice is designed to be both accessible and practical, regardless of your experience level. Moving forward, we'll explore the science of sugar addiction and strategies to overcome it.

This isn't just any book; it begins a journey toward a revitalized self. Driven by my experiences with blood sugar management and professional dedication to natural health, I aim to inspire you to take steps toward a healthier life. I invite you to embark on this journey with an open mind and dedication. Though challenging, the path leads to a healthier, more vibrant life. Together, with Sugar Defender as your ally, let's pursue a future where optimal health is not just a possibility but a reality.

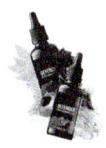

CHAPTER 1

Understanding Blood Sugar and Weight Loss.

Navigating the energy peaks and valleys throughout the day can derail even the most disciplined eating habits. This cycle isn't solely a test of willpower but is closely linked to the body's metabolic processing of food. This chapter delves into the critical role of blood sugar management in sustaining overall health and achieving effective weight loss. We simplify complex biological mechanisms, offering insights and practical advice on stabilizing blood sugar—key for pre-diabetic patients, managing type 2 diabetes, or aiming for weight loss and improved well-being.

1.1 THE SCIENCE OF BLOOD SUGAR IN WEIGHT MANAGEMENT

Understanding Glucose Metabolism Glucose is the primary energy fuel. Post-meal, food breaks down into glucose and other nutrients, absorbed into the bloodstream, prompting insulin release from the pancreas to enable cellular energy utilization. Excess glucose transforms into glycogen or fat when storage is maxed out.

This natural process regulates blood sugar and energy but also underscores the link between high sugar/carb intake and weight gain and the importance of managing glucose levels for weight control. Role of Insulin in Fat Storage Insulin facilitates glucose cell entry and aids in fat storage. With a constant surplus of glucose, insulin converts this excess into fat.

While this process is evolutionary, in today's high-calorie environment, it can lead to unwanted weight gain and insulin resistance, increasing type 2 diabetes risk and complicating weight management. Glycemic Index and Weight Control The glycemic index (GI) helps gauge food's impact on blood sugar. High-GI foods cause quick, high spikes, leading to increased hunger and potential overeating. Conversely, low-GI foods stabilize blood sugar and insulin levels, promoting satiety and aiding weight loss.

Incorporating low-GI foods into your diet supports balanced blood sugar levels and can curb the appetite. Interrelation between Blood Sugar Levels and Hunger Signals Balanced blood sugar regulates hunger hormones like ghrelin and leptin, maintaining appetite control. Fluctuating blood sugar, however, can trigger false hunger or cravings, undermining weight loss efforts. Armed with the science of blood sugar regulation, you can make informed dietary choices supporting weight stability and long-term health, moving beyond mere calorie counting.

1.2 HOW SUGAR DEFENDER HELPS STABILIZE BLOOD SUGAR.

Sugar Defender is formulated with a select blend of natural ingredients known for their positive effects on blood sugar stability, notably cinnamon, berberine, and chromium. Cinnamon is renowned for its capacity to lower blood sugar levels and increase insulin sensitivity. Berberine enhances insulin efficiency and slows carbohydrate digestion, while chromium plays a critical role in fat and carbohydrate metabolism, supporting insulin function and contributing to stable blood sugar levels.

The product works by boosting the body's natural insulin sensitivity and gradually releasing glucose, thereby avoiding sudden spikes in blood sugar that can contribute to fat accumulation and various health complications. This effect is achieved through the combined action of its ingredients, facilitating a more effective use of glucose for energy, which assists in weight management and reduces the risk of converting glucose into fat.

Unlike many conventional blood sugar management options, Sugar Defender relies on natural, non-GMO ingredients, minimizing the risk of side effects such as hypoglycemia associated with some pharmaceuticals. This holistic approach seeks to enhance the body's glucose management capabilities without adverse effects.

The effectiveness of Sugar Defender is reflected in user testimonials, such as a middle-aged teacher from Colorado who, despite prediabetes and a hectic lifestyle, experienced stabi lized blood sugar levels and increased energy after incorporating Sugar Defender into her routine along with dietary adjustments. Such accounts underscore Sugar Defender's significant potential to improve health outcomes through natural, carefully selected ingredients.

1.3 IDENTIFYING PERSONAL BLOOD SUGAR TRIGGERS

Understanding your unique blood sugar triggers is essential for managing diabetes and supporting weight loss effectively. Each person's body responds differently to foods and lifestyle habits, making it crucial to identify what specifically causes your blood sugar to spike. Common Dietary Triggers Refined carbohydrates, sugary drinks, and high-sugar snacks are well-known for causing blood sugar spikes. However, high-glycemic fruits, certain starchy vegetables, and even large portions of whole grains can also disrupt glucose levels.

Keeping a detailed food diary, noting everything you consume and any subsequent changes in your blood sugar levels, can illuminate your dietary triggers. Impact of Lifestyle Factors Lifestyle elements such as stress, sleep, and physical activity significantly affect blood sugar management. Elevated cortisol from chronic stress can increase blood sugar and insulin resistance, while poor sleep can disrupt hormones controlling blood sugar. Regular physical activity boosts insulin sensitivity. Combining stress management techniques, ensuring 7-9 hours of sleep nightly, and incorporating a balanced exercise regimen are vital steps.

Personal Monitoring Techniques Using glucose monitoring devices, like Continuous Glucose Monitors (CGMs) or traditional fingerstick meters, allows real-time tracking of how different factors affect your blood sugar. This personalized data is crucial for tailoring your diet and lifestyle to manage your diabetes better.

Adapting Diet and Lifestyle After identifying your triggers, adjust your diet and lifestyle to mitigate them. Reduce portions of problematic foods or switch to lower glycemic alternatives. Incorporate stress-reduction practices and ensure adequate rest and physical activity. These adjustments should not feel drastic but rather be mindful decisions that create a balanced, healthy lifestyle without feeling restricted. Regular monitoring as you make these changes helps maintain optimal glucose control, contributing to weight loss and overall well-being.

1.4 THE IMPACT OF UNSTABLE BLOOD SUGAR ON YOUR HEALTH

Unstable blood sugar levels can profoundly disrupt daily life, leading to physical and psychological challenges. Symptoms like fatigue, irritability, and dizziness can impair daily functioning, creating a risk, especially in situations requiring alertness, such as driving. The long-term effects of poor blood sugar management can be severe, potentially resulting in type 2 diabetes and its associated health complications, including cardiovascular diseases, diabetic neuropathy, and organ damage.

These conditions not only deteriorate physical health but also pose significant psychological strains, manifesting as anxiety and depression and impacting overall quality of life. Moreover, the social and economic implications of managing diabetes are substantial. The costs associated with medical care, medications, and potential loss of income due to health-related work absences can place a heavy financial burden on individuals.

Socially, it can lead to isolation and decreased engagement in community or family activities. Understanding the importance of stable blood sugar emphasizes the avoidance of discomfort and the necessity of maintaining overall health and well-being. Early recognition and proactive management of blood sugar levels are crucial steps toward a healthier, more balanced life.

1.5 NATURAL INGREDIENTS IN SUGAR DEFENDER AND THEIR BENEFITS.

Understanding the role of each ingredient in Sugar Defender is crucial for appreciating its benefits on blood sugar levels and metabolic health. The supplement's formula isn't a random mix but a carefully curated selection of components known for their positive effects on blood sugar regulation. Cinnamon is a key player in this supplement, long valued for its medicinal properties. It has been shown to lower fasting blood sugar and enhance insulin sensitivity, acting similarly to insulin and promoting glucose uptake into cells.

Additionally, its antioxidant properties help combat oxidative stress, which is often prevalent in those with high blood sugar. Berberine, another vital ingredient, is celebrated for its ability to reduce blood glucose levels and boost insulin sensitivity, rivaling the effectiveness of some diabetes medications. It activates the AMPK enzyme and aids in metabolism regulation and glucose absorption. Chromium, essential for metabolizing carbohydrates and fats, supports insulin activity. Research supports its role in diminishing insulin resistance and controlling blood sugar in type 2 diabetes patients.

Alpha-lipoic acid, also part of the formula, is a potent antioxidant that improves insulin sensitivity and mitigates diabetic neuropathy symptoms by shielding the nervous system. The synergistic interaction of these ingredients enhances their benefits, offering a holistic approach to blood sugar management. This combination targets blood sugar control and amplifies overall metabolic health improvements. Regarding safety, Sugar Defender's natural ingredients are generally well-tolerated, reflecting their historical use in traditional medicine.

Although the risk of side effects is minimal, consulting a healthcare provider before starting any new supplement is advisable, particularly for those with existing conditions or on medication. In comparing Sugar Defender's natural ingredients to the synthetic alternatives in the market, the former works in harmony with the body's natural functions, supporting and enhancing them without the risk of side effects or disrupting metabolic processes. This aligns with a balanced and sustainable health management approach. Opting for Sugar Defender means choosing a product designed for effective blood sugar stabilization, prioritizing safety, and aligning with the body's natural processes. Its scientifically backed, natural formulation presents it as a dependable option for managing blood sugar levels and enhancing overall health.

1.6 SETTING REALISTIC GOALS FOR BLOOD SUGAR MANAGEMENT

Effective blood sugar management hinges on setting realistic, clear, and achievable goals using the SMART framework—Specific, Measurable, Achievable, Relevant, and Time-bound. This strategic approach is designed to optimize blood sugar level control efficiently. Start by setting Specific goals. Rather than a broad objective like "I want to lower my blood sugar," aim for precise targets, such as reducing your fasting blood sugar to under 120 mg/dL.

Making your goals Measurable allows tracking progress, whether it's daily carbohydrate intake or a desired decrease in your HbA1c over a set period. Ensure your goals are Achievable, considering your current health and lifestyle. Unrealistic targets can lead to frustration and demotivation. Instead, opt for gradual improvements, acknowledging what is realistically attainable. Relevant goals should align with your overall health objectives and reasons for managing your blood sugar, encompassing regular exercise and dietary changes supporting diabetes management.

Finally, deadlines for every goal must be established to make it time-bound. This creates urgency and fosters motivation, whether reaching a specific blood sugar level in three months or committing to daily physical activity—incremental Changes Approach blood sugar stabilization as a marathon, not a sprint. Focus on small, manageable lifestyle adjustments rather than abrupt changes. Simple steps, such as swapping sugary beverages for water or incrementally increasing daily activity, can cumulatively lead to significant blood sugar improvements and are less overwhelming.

Monitoring Progress Regular blood sugar monitoring is essential for effective diabetes management. It helps gauge the success of your efforts and the impact of lifestyle changes. Adjust your goals based on monitoring outcomes to ensure they remain realistic and aligned with your health status.

Motivational Strategies Maintaining motivation is crucial. Implement short-term rewards for achieving goals and consider joining support groups for encouragement. Tracking your progress visually through graphs or charts can also serve as a potent motivator, illustrating your advancements toward a healthier life. By adhering to the SMART goals framework, embracing gradual lifestyle changes, consistently monitoring progress, and employing motivational strategies, you can effectively manage your blood sugar and enhance your overall health, steering towards a vibrant, healthier future.

Exercise caution when navigating the blood sugar management supplements market, as numerous counterfeit products mimic reputable brands, potentially jeopardizing your health. While visually similar, these imitations may lack the efficacy of genuine products and could adversely affect your blood sugar levels and diabetes management. To ensure the integrity and efficacy of your supplement, it is imperative to procure Sugar Defender directly from the official website. This measure safeguards against the risks associated with counterfeit products and guarantees that you receive a product formulated to support your health goals.

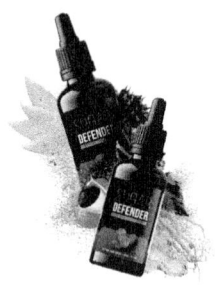

Please click the link and visit the website if you need more information. You can also order the products only from the website.

Click the link or copy and paste it into your browser.

https://hop.clickbank.net/?affiliate=hentom56&vendor=sugardef&pid=pre1

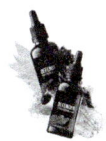

CHAPTER 2

Dietary Approaches to Support Blood Sugar Balance

Envision a world where each meal serves as a sensory delight and a foundational pillar for your well-being. Every bite pleases your taste buds and promotes stable energy and mood. This vision is not mere fantasy; it is within reach by adopting a low-glycemic index (GI) diet. This chapter delves into how a low-GI dietary approach can revolutionize your relationship with food, positioning every meal as a strategic choice to achieve balanced blood sugar levels and enhance overall health.

2.1 CRAFTING A LOW-GI MEAL PLAN FOR LONG-TERM HEALTH

Introduction to Low-GI Eating

The glycemic index (GI) is a valuable tool that categorizes foods on a scale from 0 to 100 based on their impact on blood sugar levels. Foods with a low GI score digest slower, fostering stable blood sugar and consistent energy levels. Slow digestion is crucial for weight management, as it improves appetite control, making you feel fuller for longer periods. Designing a low-GI diet and Creating a balanced low-GI meal plan is essential for harnessing these benefits. A well-structured plan should feature nutrient-dense breakfast options like steel-cut oats, which provide a slow-release form of energy. For lunches and dinners, focus on incorporating a variety of non-starchy vegetables, pairing them with low-GI carbohydrates such as quinoa, and complementing these with lean protein sources, for example, grilled chicken or fish. It's important to note that consistency in meal timing and stringent portion control are critical elements of a low-GI diet. This disciplined approach ensures that even foods on the lower GI scale do not contribute to unwanted blood sugar spikes.

Sample Meal Plans and Recipes Breakfast - Start your day with a bowl of Greek yogurt topped with a handful of walnuts and fresh berries for a refreshing mix of protein, healthy fats, and antioxidants. Lunch - Enjoy a grilled chicken salad featuring a lush array of mixed greens in a light vinaigrette. This meal perfectly balances protein, fiber, and healthy fats. Dinner - Savor a heart-healthy baked salmon, steamed broccoli, and a quinoa salad. This combination delivers omega-3 fatty acids, vitamins, and minerals. - Snack - pair an apple with a dollop of almond butter for a quick and satisfying snack. This not only curbs hunger pangs but also stabilizes blood sugar levels between meals. Adjusting for Individual Needs The low-GI diet is versatile and can be adapted to meet individual dietary requirements and preferences. For those who follow a vegetarian or vegan lifestyle, animal proteins can be substituted with plant-based sources such as lentils, chickpeas, or tofu. Monitoring your body's response to different foods and their impact on your blood sugar is a pragmatic approach to tailoring the diet to your health goals. This level of customization ensures that the low-GI diet not only aids in managing blood sugar levels but also supports overall well-being, contributing to a healthier, more energetic lifestyle.

2.2 DECIPHERING CARBOHYDRATES

Navigating the Good Versus the Bad Carbohydrates are a crucial component of our diet and pivotal in managing blood sugar levels—a key consideration for individuals with diabetes or those pursuing weight loss. These nutrients are broadly categorized into simple and complex carbohydrates, each differing in their impact on our health, especially concerning blood glucose stability.

Simple carbohydrates are absorbed rapidly into the bloodstream, causing swift increases in blood sugar levels. These carbohydrates are primarily found in processed and refined sugars, such as candy, sodas, and baked goods made with white flour. While they may offer a quick energy boost, this is often followed by a sharp decline, leading to a vicious cycle of cravings and overeating. In contrast, complex carbohydrates are broken down and metabolized much slower, resulting in a more steady and sustained energy source.

This group includes nutrient-rich whole grains like oats, barley, brown rice, and legumes like beans and lentils. These foods are invaluable for maintaining stable blood sugar levels and are essential for overall health, largely thanks to their high fiber content. Dietary fiber not only aids in digestion but also supports heart health and promotes satiety, which can significantly aid in weight management. To fully benefit from complex carbohydrates, it is advised to incorporate them alongside a variety of fiber-rich fruits and vegetables.

This approach ensures a well-rounded intake of essential nutrients while minimizing the risk of sudden blood sugar spikes. Adopting a diet abundant in complex carbohydrates and dietary fiber lays a solid foundation for achieving a leaner body, higher energy levels, and improved metabolic health. This strategy perfectly aligns with the objectives of natural, healthy weight loss, prioritizing the stability of blood glucose levels through carefully selecting beneficial carbohydrates.

2.3 THE ROLE OF FIBER IN MANAGING BLOOD SUGAR LEVELS

Dietary fiber, particularly soluble fiber, plays a pivotal role in blood sugar management. Soluble fiber is known for slowing down the absorption of sugar into the bloodstream, thereby helping to regulate blood sugar spikes after meals. This effect is crucial for individuals managing diabetes or prediabetes, as it aids in maintaining stable blood glucose levels throughout the day.

Foods rich in high-quality fiber, such as legumes, whole grains, fruits, and vegetables, are beneficial for digestion and enhance insulin sensitivity. This improvement in insulin response is vital for effectively converting glucose into energy, reducing the risk of insulin resistance—a common precursor to type 2 diabetes.

Moreover, whole grains and legumes are packed with essential nutrients that support metabolic health, further contributing to a balanced diet that can prevent sudden blood sugar fluctuations. To maximize the health benefits of dietary fiber, it is recommended to increase fiber intake gradually. This gradual approach, accompanied by sufficient water consumption, ensures the body can adjust without experiencing discomfort, such as bloating or gas, often associated with sudden high-fiber diets.

Incorporating various fiber-rich foods into daily meals supports blood sugar control and promotes a feeling of fullness, which can aid in weight management efforts. Weight loss or maintaining a healthy weight is particularly beneficial for individuals with diabetes or those at risk, as it can enhance insulin sensitivity and overall metabolic health.

Understanding and utilizing the power of dietary fiber in blood sugar management is a natural and effective strategy to improve your health, reduce the risk of diabetes, and support a sustainable weight loss journey.

2.4 OPTIMAL PROTEIN SOURCES FOR REGULATING BLOOD SUGAR

Proteins play a pivotal role in managing blood sugar levels by decelerating the digestive process. This slow digestion is crucial for preventing sudden spikes in blood sugar, thereby maintaining a steady energy flow and enhancing satiety. For individuals striving to balance their blood sugar, incorporating various high-quality protein sources into their diet is essential. Lean meats, such as chicken, turkey, and lean cuts of beef, are excellent sources of protein that can help stabilize blood sugar levels without adding excessive fat to the diet. Fish, particularly fatty types like salmon, mackerel, and sardines, not only provide high-quality protein but are also rich in omega-3 fatty acids, which have been shown to improve cardiovascular health and may assist in blood sugar regulation.

Eggs are another versatile and nutrient-dense option. They provide a complete source of protein, meaning they contain all nine essential amino acids your body needs for optimal health. Including eggs in your diet can help keep your blood sugar levels in check while supporting muscle repair and growth.

Plant-based proteins, including legumes such as beans, lentils, chickpeas, tofu, and tempeh, offer a dual advantage for managing blood sugar. These foods are rich in protein and contain dietary fiber, further aiding in slowing digestion and stabilizing blood sugar levels. Integrating these plant-based proteins into meals can also enhance dietary variety and provide essential nutrients, making them a valuable component of a blood sugar-friendly diet.

By carefully selecting and incorporating these high-quality protein sources across your meals, you can support blood sugar control and contribute to your overall health and well-being.

2.5 ESSENTIAL FATS FOR OPTIMAL HEALTH AND WEIGHT MANAGEMENT

In the journey towards achieving a healthier weight and improving overall health, understanding the types of fats to include in your diet is crucial. Incorporate sources of unsaturated fats, such as avocados, nuts, seeds, and fatty fish like salmon and mackerel, into your daily meals. These healthy fats are pivotal for enhancing insulin sensitivity—a key factor in blood sugar regulation—and play a significant role in supporting heart health. The omega-3 fatty acids found in fatty fish, in particular, are renowned for their anti-inflammatory properties, which can aid in preventing chronic diseases.

Conversely, it is advisable to limit your intake of trans fats and saturated fats. Trans fats, often found in fried foods, baked goods, and processed snacks, can increase LDL cholesterol levels ("bad" cholesterol) and lower HDL cholesterol levels ("good" cholesterol), thereby elevating the risk of heart disease. Saturated fats, prevalent in red meat and dairy products, should be consumed in moderation.

Excessive intake of saturated fats has been linked to increased insulin resistance, which can hinder your body's ability to use insulin effectively. This not only complicates blood sugar management but also contributes to the risk of developing type 2 diabetes and cardiovascular diseases.

By prioritizing unsaturated fats and reducing the consumption of trans and saturated fats, you can support your body in maintaining healthy blood sugar levels, fostering a robust metabolism, and reducing the risk of heart disease. This balanced approach to dietary fats is a cornerstone of natural health weight loss and a vital step toward a healthier, more vibrant life.

2.6 MASTERY OF FOOD LABELS: THE KEY TO UNVEILING HIDDEN SUGARS

Embarking on the path to managing blood sugar effectively demands a keen eye for decoding food labels, particularly to spotlight and avoid the trap of added sugars. Begin by prioritizing products that are either low in added sugars or entirely devoid of them. This strategic selection is fundamental in maintaining stable blood sugar levels, preventing rapid spikes that disrupt metabolic health, and paving the way for more complex health challenges.

Transitioning towards whole, unprocessed foods is a cornerstone in this journey. These natural choices lack the concealed sugars that lurk in many packaged foods, often masquerading under various names. Vigilance in identifying these hidden sugars is pivotal, as they are prime contributors to glucose fluctuation and, over time, can significantly hinder your health progress.

By delving deeper into the art of reading and interpreting food labels, you arm yourself with the knowledge to make informed choices. This expertise enables the crafting of a resilient eating plan that champions blood sugar regulation and effective weight management and enhances your overall health. Such a plan is not static; it evolves, mirroring your unique health objectives and dietary inclinations, thereby ensuring a tailored approach to meeting your wellness goals.

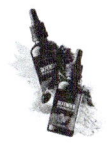

CHAPTER 3

Recipes and Meal Planning

3.1 ENERGIZING BREAKFAST IDEAS

Kickstart your day with a breakfast designed to stabilize your blood sugar levels while enhancing your metabolism. Choosing meals abundant in protein and fiber is crucial for sustaining energy levels throughout the morning and reducing the likelihood of craving unhealthy snacks. For a nutrient-packed start, consider blending a smoothie with Greek yogurt, mixed berries, a handful of spinach, and a sprinkle of ground flaxseeds. This combination offers a powerful mix of protein, fiber, and antioxidants, providing a sustained energy boost and vital nutrients to start your day.

Another excellent choice is oatmeal, which can be topped with nuts and seeds for added texture and nutrients. This meal is particularly effective in gradually releasing energy, thanks to the complex carbohydrates found in oats, which help keep blood sugar levels steady. Preparing overnight oats can be a lifesaver for those mornings when time is of the essence. Mix rolled oats with your choice of milk or a dairy-free alternative, add a touch of natural sweetener if desired, and let the mixture soften in the refrigerator overnight. Top with fresh fruit, nuts, or seeds in the morning for an extra nutrient boost.

Alternatively, assembling a Greek yogurt parfait offers another quick yet nutritious option. Layer Greek yogurt with homemade granola and fresh fruits in a glass or jar for a visually appealing and satisfying breakfast. This combination provides a rich source of protein and includes the fiber and vitamins necessary for a healthy start to the day. Integrating these energizing breakfast ideas into your routine ensures a flavorful and healthful beginning to your day, setting a positive tone for maintaining balanced blood sugar levels and a high metabolism.

3.2 BALANCED LIGHT LUNCHES

Aim for a lunch harmony of lean proteins, complex carbohydrates, and healthy fats to sidestep the common afternoon energy slump. A vibrant salad teeming with leafy greens, topped with succulently grilled chicken, and sprinkled with a handful of nuts offers a perfect blend of nutrients to keep you satiated and energized. Alternatively, a whole grain wrap cradling slices of turkey, creamy avocado, and crisp vegetables combine convenience with nutrition, making for a satisfying midday meal.

For those seeking portable yet nutritious options, mason jar salads are fantastic. Layer your favorite greens, proteins, and a drizzle of vinaigrette into a jar for a fresh grab-and-go lunch. Wraps, too, can be prepared ahead of time with various fillings such as smoked salmon, mixed greens, and a smear of hummus for a quick, healthy fix on hectic days. These light lunches are easy to prepare and ensure you're fueled with the right balance of nutrients to avoid post-lunch lethargy, keeping your metabolism humming and supporting your blood sugar management goals.

3.3 BLOOD SUGAR-FRIENDLY DINNERS

Opt for evening meals that incorporate ingredients with a low glycemic index to ensure a gentle impact on your blood sugar levels throughout the night. Dishes such as grilled salmon accompanied by roasted sweet potatoes and steamed broccoli not only provide a symphony of flavors but also deliver a balanced nutritional profile that won't cause sudden spikes in your glucose levels. Similarly, a colorful vegetable stir-fry with tofu, seasoned with herbs and a tamari sauce splash can be satisfying and beneficial for maintaining steady blood sugar.

In addition to choosing the right ingredients, practicing portion control is pivotal. You can enjoy a fulfilling dinner by serving moderate amounts without overloading your digestive system, which is particularly important in the evening. Aim to have your dinner at least three hours before sleep. This timing allows your body to adequately digest your meal, facilitating overnight blood sugar stability and a restful night's sleep. Adopting these practices for your evening meals can play a significant role in your overall blood sugar management strategy, ensuring your body is nourished, and your glucose levels remain balanced as you end your day.

3.4 SMART SNACKING STRATEGIES

To effectively manage cravings and ensure your blood sugar levels remain balanced, it's vital to select snacks that are abundant in proteins, healthy fats, and fibers. These nutrients play a key role in satiating hunger, slowing the absorption of sugar into the bloodstream, and providing a steady energy source.

Consider incorporating hummus paired with crunchy vegetables such as carrots, celery, or bell peppers for a snack that combines complex carbohydrates with proteins and healthy fats. This not only satisfies your hunger but also provides a nutrient-dense option. Alternatively, a handful of almonds or walnuts offers a portable snack that delivers protein and heart-healthy fats. It is an excellent choice for maintaining energy levels and blood sugar control.

Timing your snacks is equally important. A mid-morning snack can help bridge the gap between breakfast and lunch, preventing the temptation to overeat or choose high-sugar options due to excessive hunger. Similarly, a mid-afternoon snack can provide the energy needed to finish the day strong without succumbing to energy dips that might lead you to seek quick sugar fixes.

Including these smart snacking strategies into your daily routine can greatly assist in stabilizing blood sugar levels, managing hunger, and providing your body with the nutrients it needs to perform optimally.

3.5 GUILT-FREE DESSERTS

Embrace the joy of desserts while aligning with your health and wellness goals. By choosing natural sweeteners like stevia and monk fruit, you can relish the sweetness you desire without the adverse blood sugar spikes from traditional sugars. These natural alternatives provide the perfect solution for creating delicious and diabetes-friendly desserts.

For a refreshing and guilt-free option, consider preparing a lush berry compote. Sweeten this vibrant mix of berries with monk fruit, a natural sweetener that doesn't impact your blood sugar levels. Serve this delightful compote over a generous dollop of whipped coconut cream for a decadent treat that feels indulgent yet remains guilt-free. This dessert satisfies your sweet tooth and packs a nutritional punch with its antioxidant-rich berries and healthy fats from the coconut cream. Alternatively, if you're in the mood for something rich and chocolaty, explore a flourless chocolate cake's satisfyingly dense and moist textures. Using stevia as a sweetener makes this cake a safe indulgence that won't compromise your blood sugar management efforts. The absence of flour reduces the carbohydrate content, making it an excellent choice for those monitoring their glucose levels closely.

The secret to enjoying these desserts lies in moderation and mindful eating. Paying close attention to portion sizes and savoring each bite can dramatically enhance your dining experience. This mindful approach allows you to indulge in your favorite treats without the fear of overindulgence or the guilt that often follows. Incorporating these strategies into your dessert choices ensures you can enjoy delicious, sweet treats while maintaining a balanced diet. These guilt-free desserts support your health objectives by providing options low in sugar and high in flavor, allowing you to indulge your dessert cravings healthily and satisfyingly.

3.6 MASTERING MEAL PREPARATION

Diving into the world of meal prepping and batch cooking unlocks a pathway to maintaining a healthy lifestyle while ensuring your diet supports your blood sugar management and weight loss objectives. You can significantly streamline your dietary routine by dedicating time to planning your meals for the week, cooking in larger quantities, and utilizing the appropriate kitchen tools. This strategy not only aids in adhering to a balanced and nutritious diet but also alleviates the daily stress of meal decisions.

Begin by allocating a portion of your weekend to planning your meals for the coming week. Consider incorporating a diverse array of dishes that align with your health goals, focusing on recipes rich in lean proteins, complex carbohydrates, and healthy fats. Once your menu is set, compile a comprehensive shopping list to ensure you have all the necessary ingredients.

Batch cooking is your next step. This involves preparing multiple servings of meals at once, which can be a game-changer for your diet. Cooking large quantities of staples like quinoa, brown rice, or lean proteins can save you time during the week. Additionally, assembling and freezing soups, stews, or casseroles in individual portions creates convenient, ready-to-eat meals that require minimal effort to serve. Investing in quality storage containers that are both freezer-friendly and microwave-safe will keep your meals fresh and make reheating a breeze.

Embracing these meal preparation strategies guarantees you access to healthy, nutritious meals throughout the week and plays a crucial role in managing your blood sugar levels and supporting your weight loss journey. With a well-planned meal prep routine, you can enjoy a varied and satisfying diet that promotes your overall health and well-being, ensuring your blood sugar remains stable and your energy levels are consistent. This holistic approach to meal preparation empowers you to maintain a balanced diet, focusing on your health needs without sacrificing flavor or variety.

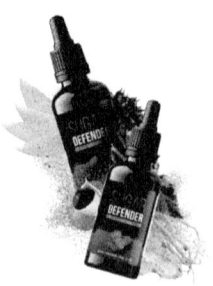

Please click the link and visit the website if you need more information. You can also order the products only from the website.

Click the link or copy and paste it into your browser.

https://hop.clickbank.net/?affiliate=hentom56&vendor=sugardef&pid=pre1

CHAPTER 4

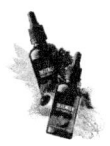

Lifestyle Modifications for Better Blood Sugar

4.1 REGULAR PHYSICAL ACTIVITY

Regular physical activity is a cornerstone for effectively managing diabetes and supporting weight management efforts. Engaging in a balanced mix of aerobic exercises, strength training, and flexibility routines is instrumental in enhancing insulin sensitivity and optimizing blood sugar levels. By incorporating these varied forms of exercise into your daily regimen, you facilitate efficient glucose metabolism and bolster your overall health and vitality.

Aerobic exercises, such as brisk walking, cycling, or swimming, are pivotal in improving cardiovascular health and blood circulation. These activities are especially beneficial for heart health, which is crucial for individuals managing diabetes. On the other hand, strength training activities, including using resistance bands, bodyweight exercises, or lifting weights, are vital for increasing muscle mass. Greater muscle mass is inherently more metabolically active, meaning it helps burn calories more efficiently and significantly regulates blood glucose levels.

In addition to aerobic and strength training, incorporating flexibility exercises like yoga or Pilates into your routine can have profound benefits on stress levels, which can positively impact blood sugar control. These practices improve flexibility and core strength and encourage mental relaxation and stress reduction, further supporting metabolic health. To cultivate a sustainable exercise regimen, it's essential to start with short, achievable sessions that suit your current fitness level and gradually build up the duration and intensity of your workouts. Striving for a well-rounded routine that includes a balance of aerobic, strength, and flexibility training each week can keep your exercise plan engaging and effective.

Monitoring your blood sugar levels before and after each exercise session can provide valuable insights into how different types of physical activity influence your glucose metabolism. This allows you to tailor your exercise plan to better meet your metabolic health needs. This personalized approach ensures that your physical activity regimen not only supports your diabetes management goals but also contributes to a healthier, more balanced lifestyle.

4.2 SLEEP: THE ESSENTIAL FOUNDATION OF BLOOD SUGAR STABILITY

Achieving and maintaining quality sleep is crucial in managing blood sugar levels and reducing the risk of type 2 diabetes. Disruptions in sleep patterns can significantly affect hormonal equilibrium, leading to elevated blood sugar levels. To combat this, establishing a consistent sleep schedule is vital. Consistency reinforces your body's sleep-wake cycle, promoting deeper, more restorative sleep.

Another critical step is creating a sleep-conducive environment. This includes optimizing bedroom temperature, minimizing noise and light exposure, and investing in comfortable mattresses and pillows. These measures collectively create an ambiance that encourages sound sleep. For those grappling with sleep disorders such as sleep apnea, seeking professional guidance is essential. Addressing and managing these conditions improves sleep quality and supports metabolic health, reducing the strain on your body's ability to regulate blood sugar effectively.

Strategies for Enhanced Sleep Quality

To further improve sleep quality, consider incorporating relaxation techniques into your evening routine. Activities such as reading, gentle yoga, or meditation can significantly help calm the mind and prepare the body for sleep. Additionally, leveraging sleep technology aids—such as white noise machines or sleep tracking devices—can offer insights into your sleep patterns and help identify areas for improvement. Emphasizing regular, quality sleep plays a pivotal role in hormonal balance and glucose metabolism, thus forming a foundational pillar in your overall health management strategy.

4.3 EFFECTIVE STRESS MANAGEMENT FOR OPTIMAL BLOOD SUGAR CONTROL

Chronic stress elevates blood sugar levels by increasing cortisol production. This hormonal surge can compromise the management of diabetes, making effective stress management techniques an essential aspect of metabolic health. Mindfulness meditation is a powerful tool in the stress management arsenal. It helps anchor the mind in the present moment and alleviate worry. Similarly, deep breathing exercises can activate the body's relaxation response, counteracting the effects of stress and leading to lower cortisol levels.

Incorporating yoga into your daily routine not only aids in stress reduction but also benefits physical health by improving flexibility, strength, and circulation. Monitoring the impact of these practices can provide valuable insights, allowing for adjustments that optimize their effectiveness in managing stress and supporting blood sugar control.

Adopting a holistic approach that includes stress management, alongside regular physical activity, adequate sleep, and careful dietary choices, creates a comprehensive strategy for maintaining optimal blood sugar levels and promoting overall well-being.t for Blood Sugar Control Chronic stress elevates blood sugar levels by increasing cortisol, which can disrupt diabetes management. Mindfulness meditation, deep breathing exercises, and yoga are effective stress reduction techniques that can lower cortisol levels and aid in blood sugar control. Integrating these practices into your daily routine and monitoring their effectiveness can improve your stress response and metabolic health.

4.4 LIFESTYLE CHOICES

Understanding the Effects of Alcohol and Smoking Moderating alcohol consumption and eliminating smoking are essential actions for those managing diabetes. Alcohol's impact on blood sugar levels can be complex and unpredictable. It can cause an immediate increase in blood sugar but also has the potential to lead to dangerously low levels hours later, especially for those on insulin or certain diabetes medications. Therefore, understanding and moderating alcohol intake is crucial to maintaining balance and avoiding these unpredictable swings. Similarly, smoking poses significant risks, exacerbating the challenges of diabetes management. It increases the body's resistance to insulin, making blood sugar control more difficult. This heightened insulin resistance elevates the risk of developing further complications associated with diabetes, including cardiovascular diseases, kidney damage, and impaired vision. Moreover, the combination of diabetes and smoking can accelerate the damage to the body's circulatory system, leading to more severe health outcomes. To navigate these challenges, adopting healthier lifestyle habits is key. For individuals looking to quit smoking, a variety of resources are available, including counseling, nicotine replacement therapies, and support groups. These tools can provide the necessary support and strategies to overcome addiction, significantly improving blood sugar control and enhancing overall health and well-being. In summary, making informed lifestyle choices regarding alcohol and smoking can have a profound impact on diabetes management. By moderating alcohol intake and seeking support to quit smoking, individuals can take significant steps toward better health, improved blood sugar stability, and a reduced risk of diabetes-related complications.

4.5 EVALUATING NATURAL SUPPLEMENTS FOR BLOOD SUGAR MANAGEMENT

In natural health, certain supplements such as cinnamon, magnesium, and alpha-lipoic acid have garnered attention for their potential benefits in regulating blood sugar levels. Cinnamon, for instance, is believed to mimic insulin's activity and increase insulin sensitivity, making it a popular choice among those looking to manage their blood sugar naturally. Magnesium plays a critical role in glucose metabolism and insulin function, with deficiencies linked to higher risks of type 2 diabetes. Alpha-lipoic acid, an antioxidant, may enhance insulin sensitivity and alleviate symptoms of diabetic neuropathy.

Despite their promising attributes, it is crucial to exercise caution when incorporating these supplements into your health regimen. The efficacy and safety of supplements can vary, and their interaction with prescribed diabetes medications may lead to unforeseen complications. Before introducing any new supplement, consultation with healthcare professionals is indispensable. This step ensures that the supplement will not only be safe in the context of your overall health condition and current medications but also effective as part of a broader diabetes management strategy.

Moreover, it is advisable to source these supplements from reputable providers to guarantee their purity and potency. The market is saturated with products of varying quality, and only high-grade supplements can provide the desired health benefits without posing risks of contamination or incorrect dosing. Incorporating natural supplements should be viewed as one component of a comprehensive approach to diabetes management that includes diet, exercise, stress reduction, and medication as a healthcare provider prescribes. By carefully evaluating and selecting natural supplements under professional guidance, individuals with diabetes can enhance their blood sugar control and overall metabolic health.

4.6 MAINTAINING MOTIVATION AND MONITORING PROGRESS

To effectively manage diabetes and support weight loss, setting realistic, achievable goals is paramount. These objectives provide direction and purpose, guiding daily actions and decisions. Equally important is the utilization of digital tools for tracking progress. Applications that monitor food intake, physical activity, blood glucose levels, and weight can offer invaluable insights into your health journey, enabling you to make informed adjustments to your lifestyle.

Celebrating milestones plays a crucial role in sustaining motivation. Recognizing achievements, no matter how small, reinforces positive behavior and fosters a sense of accomplishment. Whether maintaining blood sugar within target ranges, losing a set amount of weight, or consistently adhering to a workout regimen, each milestone deserves recognition.

Adjusting goals as needed is critical to a sustainable health management strategy. As your body changes and adapts, so too should your goals. This dynamic approach allows for a more personalized and flexible pathway to success, accommodating unforeseen challenges and obstacles that may arise. Embracing a flexible approach to challenges is essential. Obstacles are inevitable, but their impact on your progress depends on how you respond. Viewing challenges as opportunities for learning and growth can transform setbacks into stepping stones toward your goals.

These strategies collectively foster a proactive and empowered approach to diabetes management, emphasizing the importance of a balanced, health-focused lifestyle. By maintaining motivation and closely monitoring progress, you can navigate the journey of managing diabetes with confidence and resilience, ultimately achieving better health outcomes.

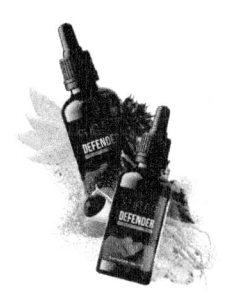

Please click the link and visit the website if you need more information. You can also order the products only from the website.

Click the link or copy and paste it into your browser.

https://hop.clickbank.net/?affiliate=hentom56&vendor=sugardef&pid=pre1

Your Feedback Could Change Lives

It is health that is real wealth and not pieces of gold and silver.

MAHATMA GANDHI

Getting a handle on blood sugar management is the key to unlocking health improvements for so many people, yet so few of us have any idea of where to start. As you can see, it's more straightforward than it sounds, but at the same time, it's quite a journey, and it requires dedication. There's no quick, easy fix. Even with Sugar Defender on your team, the best approach is still a holistic one, and managing your blood sugar requires lifestyle changes as well.

This issue is one that's personal to me, having whipped my own blood sugar levels into shape, but it's also my professional experience and having met so many people for whom this information has been life-changing that led me to write this book. Whether they're looking to lose weight, manage their diabetes, or simply live a more energetic and vibrant life, many people want to get a better handle on their blood sugar levels, and it's my goal to help them get there.

You're going to feel significant differences when you start making these changes, and that puts you in the perfect position to inspire more people to get started on this journey. You'll do this naturally by talking to others about what you've learned, but you can take it a step further and reach even more people by taking a few minutes to write a short review.

By leaving a review of this book on Amazon, you'll help new readers to find the natural, holistic, and effective approach they're looking for.

Reviews make books more visible to the audiences they're designed for, and just a few sentences from you could make all the difference to someone else's life.

Thank you so much for your support. This knowledge is too good not to share!

Scan the QR code or follow this link to leave a review:

https://www.amazon.com/review/create-review/?asin=B0DBD3RGS1

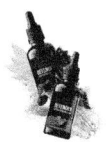

CHAPTER 5
Overcoming Challenges and Common Obstacles

5.1 OVERCOMING SUGAR CRAVINGS

Understanding the root causes of sugar cravings is essential for addressing them effectively. These cravings often arise from a complex interplay of physiological needs, such as blood sugar fluctuations, and psychological desires, which can be linked to emotional states, such as stress or boredom. Recognizing these triggers is the first step toward managing them.

To combat these cravings, consider incorporating healthy alternatives that can satisfy the sweet tooth without leading to a spike in blood sugar levels. Fresh fruits paired with nut butter offer a delightful combination of natural sugars, healthy fats, and proteins, which can help stabilize blood sugar and provide sustained energy. Similarly, Greek yogurt mixed with berries provides a creamy, sweet treat rich in protein and antioxidants, aiding blood sugar management and offering nutritional benefits.

Adopting behavioral strategies plays a crucial role in managing sugar cravings. Mindful eating encourages you to pay full attention to the eating experience, helping to identify true hunger cues and differentiate them from emotional eating. When a craving strikes, try waiting five minutes before giving in. This brief pause can often diminish the intensity of the craving, allowing you to make a more conscious decision about what you eat.

Another effective strategy is to gradually adjust your diet to minimize the intake of high-glycemic foods, which cause rapid spikes in blood sugar. Instead, focus on increasing your intake of foods high in fiber, protein, and healthy fats. Fiber helps slow down the absorption of sugar into the bloodstream, preventing sudden spikes in blood sugar that can lead to cravings. Protein and healthy fats, on the other hand, can help keep you feeling full and satisfied, reducing the likelihood of succumbing to sugar cravings.

By combining these dietary adjustments with behavioral strategies, you can effectively manage sugar cravings, supporting your metabolic health and contributing to your overall well-being.

5.2 NAVIGATING DINING OUT

Dining out presents unique challenges for managing blood sugar levels, but with a strategic approach, it can be a delightful and health-conscious experience. When perusing the menu, prioritize dishes abundant in vegetables, lean proteins, and whole grains. These selections help stabilize blood sugar and promote satiety.

Don't hesitate to inquire about how dishes are prepared. Opting for steamed, baked, or grilled meals over fried alternatives can significantly reduce unnecessary fats and calories. If a menu item interests you but is prepared in a way that doesn't align with your dietary goals, request modifications. Chefs are typically willing to accommodate such requests, allowing you to enjoy your meal without compromising your health objectives.

Portion control is another vital aspect of dining out. Restaurant portions can be generously oversized, leading to inadvertent overeating. A practical strategy is ordering starters as your main course or sharing a larger dish with a dining companion. This approach not only helps manage portion sizes but also allows you to sample a variety of flavors and nutrients.

Sauces and dressings can be hidden sources of added sugars and calories. Asking for these on the side gives you the control to determine how much—if any—to use. This simple action can drastically reduce the intake of unnecessary sugars and fats, helping you stay within your nutritional boundaries.

Adopting these mindful eating strategies allows you to enjoy dining out without compromising your blood sugar management and overall health.

5.3 NAVIGATING SOCIAL AND HOLIDAY EATING

Navigating social gatherings and holiday festivities presents unique challenges for those managing sugar intake and diabetes and striving for weight loss. To maintain your health goals during these events, it's beneficial to communicate your dietary needs in advance. When attending social gatherings, consider offering to bring a dish that aligns with your dietary regimen. This proactive approach ensures you can enjoy at least one item on the menu without compromising your health goals.

Before heading to an event, eating a well-balanced meal can significantly curb hunger, reducing the temptation to overindulge in sweets or high-calorie foods. This strategy allows you to make healthier choices and enjoy the social experience without the guilt. Holidays often revolve around food, making it a particularly challenging time to stick to dietary goals. Planning is key. Allow yourself some indulgences, but do so mindfully. Balance your plate with various vegetables, lean proteins, and moderate carbohydrates.

These foods can help stabilize blood sugar levels and keep you feeling full and satisfied. Additionally, staying active during the holiday season can counterbalance increased calorie intake and keep your metabolism engaged. Incorporate walks, family games, or any form of physical activity into your holiday traditions to maintain your health and well-being. By adopting these strategies, you can confidently navigate social and holiday eating, maintaining your health goals while still enjoying the festive spirit and camaraderie of these occasions.

5.4 BREAKING THROUGH WEIGHT LOSS PLATEAUS

Hitting a weight loss plateau can be a frustrating experience, but it's a common part of the journey toward achieving a healthier weight. The first step in breaking through a plateau is to analyze your eating habits meticulously. Keeping a detailed food diary can illuminate hidden sources of calories or reveal if your portion sizes have slowly increased. This self-monitoring can provide invaluable insights into your dietary patterns and help pinpoint areas for improvement.

To reinvigorate your metabolism and escape the monotony that accompanies long-term dieting, consider diversifying your diet with new foods and nutrients. Introducing a variety of healthy foods prevents dietary boredom and can also ensure you're receiving a full spectrum of vitamins, minerals, and antioxidants essential for optimal health and weight management.

Carefully adjusting your caloric intake and the balance of macronutrients—proteins, carbohydrates, and fats—can also play a pivotal role in overcoming a weight loss plateau. Small, strategic changes in your diet can reignite your body's fat-burning capability. For example, increasing your protein intake can boost metabolism and reduce appetite, making it easier to consume fewer calories without feeling hungry.

However, nutrition is not a one-size-fits-all science, and what works for one person may not work for another. Seeking advice from a nutrition professional can provide personalized dietary strategies tailored to your needs, preferences, and health goals. A registered dietitian or nutritionist can offer expert guidance on adjusting your diet to respect your body's unique requirements, helping you break through the plateau and continue on your path to a healthier, slimmer body.

5.5 COPING WITH SETBACKS

Setbacks are inevitable in any health and weight loss journey. Rather than viewing them as insurmountable obstacles, it's essential to embrace these moments as valuable learning opportunities that can inform and refine your strategies moving forward. Developing a mindset that accepts setbacks as part of the natural ebb and flow of progress is crucial. This approach allows you to analyze what led to the setback, identify potential triggers, and adjust your plans to better suit your needs and goals.

Setting realistic expectations is another cornerstone of effectively coping with setbacks. Unrealistic goals can lead to frustration and demotivation, particularly when progress doesn't occur at the anticipated pace or in the expected manner. By establishing achievable, incremental objectives, you create a framework for success that can be adjusted as needed, ensuring your motivation remains high and your journey towards better health continues unimpeded.

Cultivating a positive outlook is equally important. This includes practicing self-compassion, acknowledging your efforts, and recognizing your progress, no matter how small. Celebrating these small victories not only boosts your morale but also fosters resilience, making it easier to bounce back from setbacks. Additionally, this positivity helps to maintain a balanced perspective, reminding you that the path to a healthier lifestyle is a marathon, not a sprint and that every step forward counts.

Moreover, it's helpful to view setbacks not as failures but as opportunities to strengthen your commitment to your health goals. Each challenge encountered is a chance to deepen your understanding of what works best for your body and lifestyle, enabling you to make more informed decisions and tailor your approach to better suit your long-term objectives.

In summary, navigating setbacks effectively requires a blend of realistic goal setting, a positive mindset, and the flexibility to adapt strategies as needed. By viewing each setback as a stepping stone rather than a roadblock, you can maintain your motivation and progress toward a healthier, more balanced life.

5.6 SUCCESSFULLY OVERCOMING THE HURDLES OF SUGAR CRAVINGS.

Making wise choices when dining out, handling the temptations of social and holiday gatherings, breaking through weight loss stagnation, and recovering from occasional setbacks requires a comprehensive strategy that integrates thoughtful dietary decisions, deliberate behavioral modifications, and a resilient, positive attitude. By adopting these multifaceted approaches, you enable yourself to steadfastly pursue your health goals, manage diabetes with confidence, and navigate the complexities of achieving and maintaining weight loss sustainably.

Incorporating mindful eating practices helps recognize and honor your body's hunger signals and satiety cues, preventing overindulgence and supporting blood sugar regulation. Intentional behavioral changes, such as planning meals and choosing physical activities you enjoy, promote consistency and prevent boredom in your routine. Cultivating a resilient mindset prepares you to face challenges head-on and view setbacks not as failures but as opportunities for growth and learning.

Together, these strategies bolster your determination to live a healthier life. By consistently applying these principles, you strengthen your resolve and build a foundation for lasting well-being. This approach not only ensures you can manage diabetes more effectively but also empowers you to make progress toward your weight loss goals with confidence. As you continue this journey, you'll find that these combined efforts lead to a more balanced, energetic, and fulfilling lifestyle, ultimately securing your long-term success.

OVERCOMING CHALLENGES AND COMMON OBSTACLES

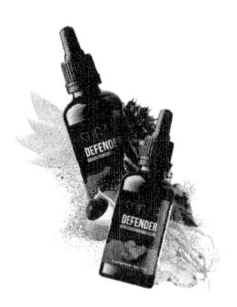

Please click the link and visit the website if you need more information. You can also order the products only from the website.

Click the link or copy and paste it into your browser.

https://hop.clickbank.net/?affiliate=hentom56&vendor=sugardef&pid=pre1

CHAPTER 6

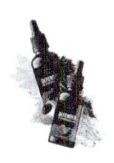

Success Stories and Motivational Insights

Imagine a life where each decision propels you towards health and vitality. This chapter honors those who've mastered their blood sugar, shed weight, and transformed their lifestyles, emerging empowered and healthier. Their stories, blueprints for a healthier life, share hope, inspiration, and practical wisdom for embracing wellness.

6.1 FROM PRE-DIABETIC TO EMPOWERED: JOHN'S JOURNEY

John, a 58-year-old dedicated high school principal, encountered a pivotal moment in his life following a prediabetes diagnosis. Faced with the daunting risk of developing type 2 diabetes, he was determined to reclaim his health. John embarked on a transformative journey, meticulously overhauling his diet to prioritize low-glycemic, nutrient-dense foods. He swapped fast food for various whole grains, lean proteins, and abundant fresh vegetables. Breakfasts became a delightful mix of oatmeal adorned with almonds and berries, while lunches and dinners featured balanced, nutritious plates rich in colors and flavors.

Once a chore, physical activity transformed into a source of joy and rejuvenation. John found solace and excitement in a new routine that included brisk walks, leisurely cycling, and refreshing swims. These activities were not just exercises but became a celebration of movement, deeply integrating into his everyday life.

The journey was not solitary. John's transformation was buoyed by an unwavering support system composed of his family, colleagues, and a dedicated healthcare team. This circle of support was instrumental in fostering sustainable lifestyle changes, providing encouragement and accountability every step of the way.

These concerted efforts bore fruit, leading to a normalization of John's blood sugar levels, effectively reversing his prediabetes. The benefits extended beyond blood sugar regulation, manifesting in significant weight loss, enhanced sleep quality, and increased energy levels. John's story is a testament to the pivotal role of dietary choices, consistent physical activity, and the strength of support networks in proactive health management. Through his journey, John transformed his health and became a beacon of hope and inspiration for others facing similar challenges.

6.2 LOSING WEIGHT AND GAINING ENERGY: LISA'S STORY

Lisa, a mother of two, overcame fatigue and excess weight by revamping her diet and exercise routine. She minimized processed foods and embraced balanced, nutrient-rich meals. Her diet focused on vegetables, lean proteins, and whole grains, controlling portion sizes to manage calorie intake. Lisa found joy in physical activities like walking, jogging, and yoga, gradually building a sustainable exercise habit. Her family supported Lisa's weight loss; she now enjoys an energetic, active lifestyle.

6.3 MANAGING TYPE 2 DIABETES

Naturally: Michael's Success Diagnosed with Type 2 Diabetes at 45,

Michael sought natural methods to manage his condition. He adopted a whole-food diet, exercised regularly, and practiced stress management. Michael tracked his blood sugar levels using a continuous glucose monitor, adjusting his lifestyle and medication with his healthcare provider's guidance.

These changes improved his blood sugar control, reduced his medication needs, and enhanced his overall health, demonstrating the impact of lifestyle changes on managing diabetes.

6.4 A FAMILY'S JOURNEY TO BETTER HEALTH

A routine doctor's visit revealed high blood sugar levels in both parents, prompting a family-wide lifestyle overhaul. Swapping takeout for home-cooked meals rich in whole ingredients, the family embraced cooking and eating together. They also became more active, enjoying walks, hikes, and community exercise. These changes led to weight loss, increased energy, and closer family bonds, illustrating the power of collective action and support in health transformation.

6.5 OVERCOMING PCOS AND INSULIN RESISTANCE: ANNA'S TALE

Anna managed her PCOS and insulin resistance by adopting a holistic approach, focusing on diet, exercise, and supplementation. A diet low in processed sugars and a cardiovascular and strength training exercise routine improved her insulin sensitivity and contributed to healthy weight loss. Supported by healthcare providers and PCOS support groups, Anna regained control over her health, underscoring the effectiveness of a holistic approach to managing health conditions.

6.6 THE ROLE OF COMMUNITY SUPPORT IN SUCCESSFUL

Health Transformation Community support is crucial in health transformation, offering motivation, accountability, and a sense of belonging. Whether online forums, local meetups, or personal networks, community support provides practical advice and encouragement. Sharing experiences and celebrating victories, big and small, are vital for sustaining long-term health changes. Success stories within these communities inspire and prove the transformative power of support in achieving and maintaining health goals. As we move forward, the journey of health transformation is enriched by the lessons and support from our communities, emphasizing that while individual actions start the path to better health, collective support ensures its sustainability and success.

CHAPTER 7

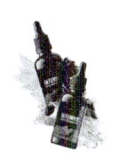

Advanced Strategies for Blood Sugar Management

Daily decisions, from meals at home to choices at social gatherings, significantly influence our health. For individuals managing diabetes and striving for weight loss, these decisions extend beyond taste, affecting blood sugar levels and overall health. This chapter delves into Intermittent Fasting (IF), a method that shifts the focus from what you eat to when you eat. IF has gained attention for its potential to transform eating habits without altering diet content. We'll examine how IF works, its benefits, and how it can be adapted to fit your lifestyle, helping you determine if it's a suitable strategy for your health objectives.

7.1 INTERMITTENT FASTING: IS IT RIGHT FOR YOU?

Intermittent fasting (IF) provides multiple protocols to align with various lifestyles and health objectives. The popular 16/8 method restricts eating to an 8-hour window, usually midday to evening, supporting social meal schedules.

Alternatively, the 5:2 diet allows regular eating for five days with a significant calorie reduction on two non-consecutive days. For those seeking a more rigorous approach, the Eat-Stop-Eat plan involves 24-hour fasts weekly.

IF offers notable benefits for blood sugar management, enhancing insulin sensitivity, and encouraging the body to utilize fat for energy. This shift can support weight loss, which is vital for managing or preventing type 2 diabetes and aiding in overall blood sugar stabilization. However, adopting IF may present hurdles such as hunger management, maintaining social eating habits, and integrating exercise. Strategies include consuming zero-calorie beverages, flexible eating windows, and customizing physical activity.

Before embarking on IF, it's essential to consider personal health conditions, particularly for individuals with diabetes or those using medications like insulin, due to the risk of hypoglycemia. Consulting with a healthcare provider ensures a tailored approach, considering the individual's age, activity level, and metabolic health. Reflective journaling can be beneficial for determining if IT suits your lifestyle. Track your eating patterns, hunger signals, cravings, and energy levels for a week. This practice can reveal insights into customizing IF to your health goals and preferences, potentially enhancing dietary habits and metabolic health.

7.2 THE KETO DIET AND BLOOD SUGAR CONTROL

The ketogenic, or keto, diet marks a dramatic departure from conventional high-carb diets recommended for diabetes management, focusing on a significant increase in fat intake and a decrease in carbohydrates. This diet shifts your body into ketosis, a metabolic state where fat, rather than glucose, is burned for energy. The typical nutrient distribution consists of 70% to 80% of calories from fat, 15% to 20% from protein, and 5% to 10% from carbohydrates, encouraging efficient fat-burning and ketone production for brain energy.

Achieving ketosis fundamentally changes your energy metabolism, moving from glucose to fat reserves for fuel. This shift has a notable effect on insulin and blood sugar levels, minimizing the spikes in blood sugar and reducing insulin needs. This is particularly beneficial for those with insulin resistance, a hallmark of type 2 diabetes, potentially improving insulin sensitivity over time. However, caution is advised for anyone on diabetes medications, as adjustments may be necessary under medical supervision.

Transitioning to a ketogenic lifestyle may initially present challenges, such as the keto flu, characterized by symptoms like headache, fatigue, and nausea, mainly due to electrolyte imbalances from reduced insulin levels. Mitigating these effects involves maintaining hydration, replenishing electrolytes, and gradually reducing carbohydrate intake to ease the body into ketosis.

A long-term ketogenic diet requires planning to ensure nutritional balance and avoid deficiencies. Incorporating nutrient-dense, low-carb vegetables and considering supplements for excluded nutrients is essential. Successful adaptation to the keto lifestyle demands a well-rounded approach to meal planning and an understanding of nutritional needs, alongside managing ketosis side effects.

Embracing the ketogenic diet as a sustainable lifestyle can enhance overall metabolic health and blood sugar control. It's important to consult healthcare professionals to customize the diet to your health needs, ensuring a safe and beneficial transition.

7.3 ADVANCED CARB COUNTING FOR FINE-TUNED CONTROL

Advanced Carb Counting and Glycemic Awareness for Blood Sugar Stability

Mastering carbohydrate management is essential for anyone striving to achieve or maintain healthy blood sugar levels, particularly for individuals with diabetes. Beyond basic carb counting, incorporating advanced strategies can greatly improve your ability to manage your blood sugar. Advanced carb counting involves accounting for the effects of dietary fiber and sugar alcohols—while fiber is a carbohydrate that doesn't convert to glucose and, therefore, doesn't spike blood sugar levels, sugar alcohols impact blood sugar less than standard sugars. By subtracting the fiber grams from total carbs and understanding that only a portion of sugar alcohol affects blood glucose, you can more accurately manage your carbohydrate intake.

Utilizing the Glycemic Index and Load for Better Meal Planning

Understanding the glycemic index (GI) and glycemic load (GL) can revolutionize your approach to managing diabetes. The GI ranks how quickly food increases blood sugar but doesn't consider serving size. The GL, however, provides a fuller picture by accounting for how much carbohydrate is in a serving of food and how much each gram of carbohydrate raises blood sugar levels. Integrating GI and GL into your diet can help you make smarter choices about the carbs you consume, tailoring your diet to minimize blood sugar spikes.

Leveraging Technology for Carb Management

The rise of digital tools has simplified tracking and managing carbohydrate intake. Carbohydrate counting apps can automatically calculate the GI and GL of foods, making it simpler to log meals and understand their impact on blood sugar levels. These apps often feature barcode scanning, which instantaneously accesses nutritional information, and meal logging integrated with blood glucose tracking to offer insights into how specific foods affect your blood sugar.

Success Stories Through Advanced Carb Management

Clara, managing type 1 diabetes, found that focusing on the glycemic load and utilizing a carb management app could stabilize her blood sugar levels more effectively, gaining insights into her dietary patterns. Similarly, Dan, who faced prediabetes, reversed his condition by monitoring his diet with an app, choosing foods based on their GI, and adjusting his carb intake to maintain healthy blood sugar levels.

Personalizing Your Fitness Routine

Creating a fitness routine that aligns with your health and fitness levels can profoundly affect your blood sugar management. Begin by assessing your cardiovascular fitness, strength, and flexibility to set realistic and personalized fitness goals. Monitoring how different exercises impact your blood sugar levels is crucial, as aerobic and strength training may affect individuals differently. Various exercises, including strength training to improve insulin sensitivity and flexibility exercises to enhance circulation, can optimize blood sugar control. Adjusting your fitness goals based on progress can help maintain motivation and ensure long-term adherence to a healthier lifestyle. In summary, integrating advanced carbohydrate counting, understanding the glycemic index and load, utilizing digital tracking tools, and personalizing your fitness routine can provide a comprehensive approach to managing diabetes and stabilizing blood sugar levels. This multifaceted strategy empowers individuals to make informed dietary and lifestyle choices, leading to improved health and well-being.

7.4 SUPPLEMENTS AND HERBS: A DEEPER DIVE

Sugar Defender

Sugar Defender product that contains a proprietary blend of 8 natural superfoods designed to rapidly target and stabilize blood sugar.

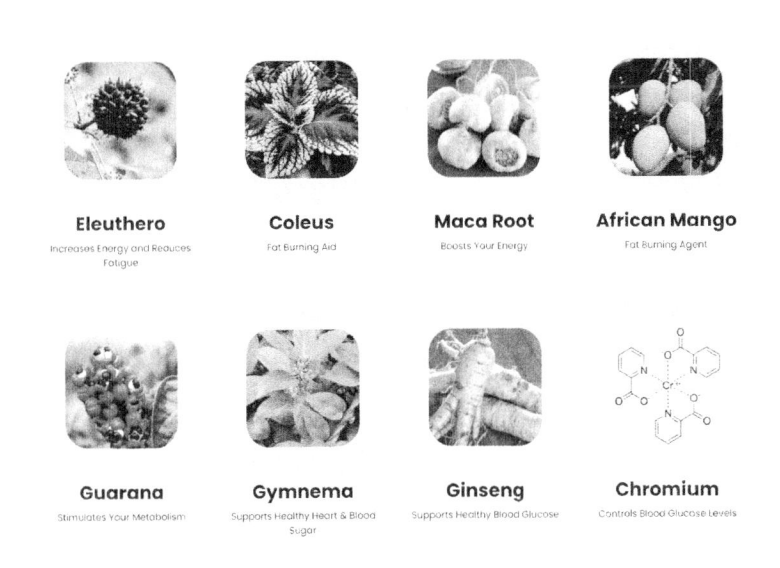

Eleuthero
Increases Energy and Reduces Fatigue

Coleus
Fat Burning Aid

Maca Root
Boosts Your Energy

African Mango
Fat Burning Agent

Guarana
Stimulates Your Metabolism

Gymnema
Supports Healthy Heart & Blood Sugar

Ginseng
Supports Healthy Blood Glucose

Chromium
Controls Blood Glucose Levels

Step 1: Eleuthero

The Adaptogenic Anchor

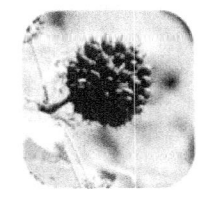

Eleuthero, often termed Siberian Ginseng, anchors the Sugar Defender formula with its adaptogenic prowess. Renowned for its ability to fortify the body's stress response and boost endurance, Eleuthero also plays a crucial role in enhancing insulin sensitivity, laying a strong foundation for blood sugar stability.

Step 2: Coleus

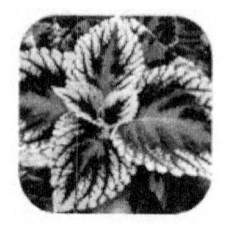

The Metabolic Enhancer

Coleus forskohlii steps in as the metabolic enhancer of the blend, thanks to its active compound, forskolin. By promoting the release of insulin and facilitating glucose's cellular uptake, Coleus works in tandem with Eleuthero, ensuring that Sugar Defender users experience a balanced metabolic rhythm.

Step 3: Maca Root

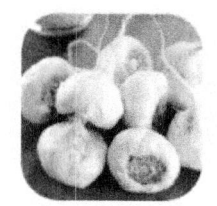

The Hormonal Harmonizer

Maca Root brings its hormone-balancing virtues to the Sugar Defender ensemble, addressing the endocrine aspect of blood sugar management. Its influence on insulin regulation is a testament to the holistic approach of Sugar Defender, ensuring that every facet of blood sugar control is addressed.

Step 4: African Mango

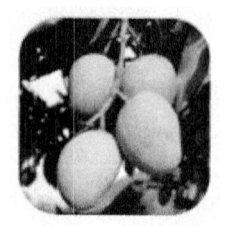

The Leptin Leverage

Integrating African Mango into the sugar-defender formula introduces a strategic leverage over leptin sensitivity. This inclusion not only aids in appetite regulation but also supports a nuanced approach to insulin resistance, highlighting the multifaceted strategy of Sugar Defender.

Step 5: Guarana

The Vigor Vitalizer

Guarana injects a burst of vitality into the Sugar Defender blend with its natural caffeine content. This component is carefully calibrated to provide an energy lift without compromising blood sugar levels, embodying the product's commitment to sustained, natural energy.

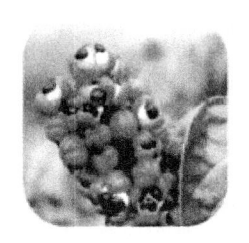

Step 6: Gymnema

The Glucose Guardian

Gymnema Sylvestre, revered as the "sugar destroyer," fortifies the Sugar Defender formula with its direct support for pancreatic health. By aiding insulin-producing cells, Gymnema underlines the product's targeted approach to maintaining glucose balance.

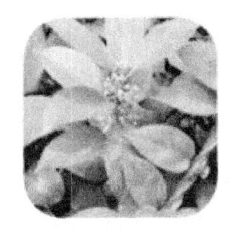

Step 7: Ginseng

The Insulin Sensitizer

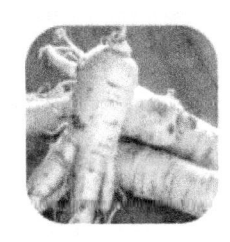

Ginseng, with its proven track record in energy enhancement and immune support, also brings insulin-sensitizing capabilities to the mix. This addition ensures that Sugar Defender users enjoy not only immediate vitality but also long-term metabolic health.

Step 8: Chromium

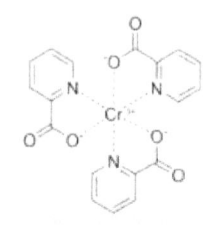

The Glucose Optimizer

Rounding off the Sugar Defender formula, Chromium acts as the essential mineral for optimal glucose metabolism. It reinforces the action of insulin, ensuring that every drop of Sugar Defender contributes to a stable and efficient blood sugar regulation.

Other supplements and herbs can help you with sugar problems and diabetes.

Berberine stands out as a potent plant extract, notable for its ability to lower blood sugar levels in type 2 diabetes by activating the AMPK enzyme, enhancing glucose utilization. Comparable in efficacy to metformin, berberine's recommended dosage is 900 to 1500 mg daily, divided into three doses with meals to minimize side effects.

Omega-3 fatty acids, though primarily known for heart health, also improve insulin sensitivity and blood sugar regulation. Opting for fish oil supplements can increase omega-3 intake, but selecting mercury-free products is crucial.

Bitter melon, akin to insulin in its action, can be consumed as a vegetable or supplement to help reduce blood sugar levels. Due to its potency, please consult a healthcare provider to ensure it doesn't interfere with your diabetes medication. Personalizing supplement and herb intake, in consultation with healthcare professionals, is key to safely enhancing your diabetes management and overall health.

Ceylon Cinnamon

Ceylon Cinnamon, also known as true cinnamon, is derived from the inner bark of the Cinnamomum verum tree. It has a long history of traditional use for its potential health benefits, including blood sugar control. This ingredient is also present in the VI authority Berberine supplement, known for helping maintain healthy blood sugar levels.

A 2010 study by J Diabetes Sci Technol suggests that Ceylon Cinnamon may improve insulin sensitivity. The study further suggests that Ceylon may enhance glucose uptake by cells, and inhibit certain enzymes involved in glucose metabolism. These mechanisms can potentially contribute to better blood sugar regulation.

Alpha Lipoic Acid (ALA)

Alpha-Lipoic Acid is a natural compound that functions as a powerful antioxidant in the body. It is involved in energy metabolism and can help regenerate other antioxidants, such as vitamins C and E, as we described in our Ami clear Review article.

A 2022 study published on Nutrients showed that alpha-lipoic acid may improve insulin sensitivity, enhance glucose uptake by cells, and reduce oxidative stress and inflammation associated with diabetes. These properties make it a potential candidate for supporting blood sugar control.

When incorporating these supplements, be mindful of potential interactions with existing medications. Berberine, for instance, may affect blood sugar levels to the point of hypoglycemia if combined with diabetes medications. Similarly, chromium could interact with insulin and other diabetes drugs, necessitating dosage adjustments. Always consult your healthcare provider before starting any new supplement to ensure a harmonious addition to your treatment plan.

Herbal remedies like cinnamon, celebrated for its flavor and blood sugar-lowering properties, can increase insulin sensitivity. A dose of 1 to 6 grams daily is typical, but caution is advised for those on blood-thinning medications. Fenugreek seeds, rich in soluble fiber, improve insulin function and slow carbohydrate absorption. 5 to 30 grams per meal is recommended for blood sugar control. Start with a lower dose to minimize gastrointestinal side effects.

7.5 The Future of Blood Sugar Management Technology

At the intersection of technology and healthcare, diabetes management is witnessing a transformative revolution. Advanced technologies like continuous glucose monitors (CGMs), insulin pumps, and artificial pancreas systems are making significant strides in how individuals monitor and manage their condition. These technologies enhance quality of life and simplify diabetes care complexities.

CGMs revolutionize diabetes management by offering real-time glucose level insights, essential for informed decisions regarding diet, exercise, and insulin use. These devices, inserted under the skin, continuously track glucose in interstitial fluid, transmitting data to monitors or smartphone apps. This continuous monitoring is pivotal in identifying glucose level patterns and preventing hypo and hyperglycemic events. Moreover, CGMs' integration with insulin pumps has led to the development of artificial pancreas systems, automating insulin delivery and significantly easing the decision-making process for those with diabetes. Artificial Intelligence (AI) plays a crucial role in diabetes management. Algorithms analyze CGM data to identify patterns and predict glucose trends. This allows for a customized management approach, potentially minimizing the risk of complications due to unstable blood sugar levels. Recent insulin delivery innovations, including inhalable insulin and microneedle patches, offer less invasive and more user-friendly alternatives to traditional injection methods. These developments promise a less intimidating experience for insulin therapy. However, these technologies' benefits are tempered by challenges with access and affordability. The high costs of CGMs, insulin pumps, novel insulin delivery systems, and inconsistent insurance coverage create financial barriers for many. Addressing these challenges involves advocating for better insurance coverage, reducing diabetes supply costs, and supporting underserved populations.

The evolution of diabetes management technology aims to improve individual health outcomes and overhaul the broader approach to diabetes care. By integrating advanced technologies, individuals can manage their diabetes with unprecedented precision and personalization, moving towards more proactive and preventive care models. This approach can potentially mitigate long-term diabetes complications and significantly enhance the quality of life.

Looking ahead, the future of blood sugar management will focus on leveraging technology to develop more integrated, personalized, and accessible diabetes care solutions. Innovations will continue to prioritize enhancing health outcomes and tackling access and affordability issues, ensuring that transformative technologies benefit everyone affected by diabetes. The next chapter delves into the personal stories of individuals who have harnessed these technologies, offering insights into the tangible impacts of these advancements in diabetes care.

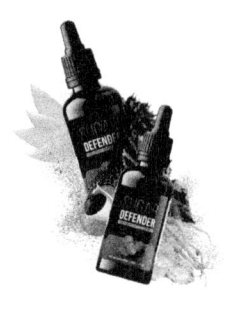

Please click the link and visit the website if you need more information. You can also order the products only from the website.

Click the link or copy and paste it into your browser.

https://hop.clickbank.net/?affiliate=hentom56&vendor=sugardef&pid=pre1

CHAPTER 8

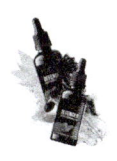

Maintaining Your Gains and Preventing Relapse

As the sun rises on the horizon, marking the beginning of a new day, it's a powerful reminder of the daily renewal and the continuous effort required to maintain the health strides you've achieved. For many, reaching their health goals—stabilizing blood sugar, managing diabetes, or shedding unwanted pounds—is a monumental feat. However, the true challenge often lies not in reaching these goals but in maintaining them long-term and preventing any backslide. This chapter is dedicated to turning your hard-won gains into a sustainable lifestyle, ensuring that your progress becomes a permanent part of your journey.

8.1 SETTING UP A LONG-TERM MAINTENANCE PLAN

Developing a Sustainable Lifestyle Blueprint Crafting a sustainable lifestyle blueprint is essential for long-term health. It requires a holistic approach that includes diet, physical activity, and mental health. The blueprint should be comprehensive, addressing nutritional needs and incorporating regular exercise, yet flexible enough to adapt to life's changes.

Reassess dietary habits frequently, ensuring a balanced diet that maintains stable blood sugar levels. As life evolves, adjust your diet to reflect activity level, age, or health changes. Incorporate nutrient-rich foods to prevent nutritional deficiencies and maintain interest in your meals. Physical activity is crucial; aim for a balanced mix of cardiovascular, strength, and flexibility exercises tailored to your fitness level and health goals. Managing stress is equally important, as chronic stress can undermine diet and exercise efforts and affect blood sugar and overall health. Regularly engage in stress-reduction practices like yoga, meditation, or deep-breathing exercises.

Importance of Routine Establishing a routine is key to sustaining a healthy lifestyle. Convert deliberate choices into habits, integrating meal planning, scheduling grocery shopping, and regular exercise into your daily life. A solid routine reduces the effort needed to make healthy choices.

Flexibility in Maintenance However, maintain flexibility to adapt your health plan as needed, responding to new health issues, changes in personal circumstances, or shifts in interest. The objective is to find sustainable practices that suit your evolving lifestyle.

Role of Periodic Reassessment: Periodically reassess your maintenance plan to ensure it meets your needs. Review your diet, exercise, and stress management strategies every few months to align with any new health goals. Utilize blood sugar tracking, fitness apps, or journaling to monitor progress and pinpoint areas for improvement.

Embrace a maintenance mindset focused on continuously adapting your lifestyle practices to meet changing needs, ensuring your health management is a lifelong journey toward well-being. With the right strategies, your progress marks the beginning of enduring health and happiness.

8.2 REGULAR CHECK-UPS AND WHEN TO SEEK PROFESSIONAL HELP

Maintaining health gains, especially when managing blood sugar or weight, demands consistent self-care and regular check-ups. Annual health evaluations are vital to identify potential issues early and adjust health plans accordingly. These check-ups should include physical exams and comprehensive blood tests, like lipid profiles and liver function tests. For those with diabetes, monitoring A1C levels every three to six months is crucial to assess blood sugar control over time.

Monitoring blood pressure and cardiovascular health is essential, as diabetes heightens the risk of heart issues. Regular screenings can detect early changes, allowing for timely interventions. Eye health screenings are also recommended to prevent complications like diabetic retinopathy. Being aware of warning signs is crucial. Noticeable changes such as unexplained weight shifts, frequent infections, or persistent fatigue could signal the need for professional evaluation. These symptoms might indicate blood sugar fluctuations, immune system issues, or other health imbalances.

Effective management often requires assembling a diverse healthcare team, including a primary care physician, an endocrinologist, a dietitian, and possibly a diabetes educator. Mental health support can also play a significant role in managing the emotional challenges of living with chronic conditions.

Navigating healthcare services effectively is key. Prepare for appointments by noting symptoms, questions, and current medications. Advocacy is important—speak up about concerns or when you need clarification on treatment plans. Keeping detailed records of medical interactions can aid in tracking progress and facilitating informed care decisions.

Regular check-ups and a supportive healthcare team are fundamental to sustaining health improvements. Proactively engaging with healthcare services and building a comprehensive support system ensures ongoing health and well-being.

8.3 EDUCATING FRIENDS AND FAMILY ON YOUR LIFESTYLE CHOICES

Embarking on a journey to better manage your health, especially concerning blood sugar and weight, requires the understanding and support of those closest to you. Effectively communicating the importance of these lifestyle changes is crucial for your well-being. Begin by explaining that stabilizing blood sugar through diet is not solely about weight loss but also about preventing severe health issues associated with unmanaged diabetes, such as heart disease and vision loss. Use simple analogies, like comparing a balanced diet to high-quality fuel for a car, to clarify why you prefer whole, unprocessed foods.

Friends and family often resist due to misconceptions about diabetes and dietary management. Tackle these conversations with empathy, acknowledging that your lifestyle changes might challenge their traditional views on meals and family gatherings. If skepticism arises, offer resources or suggest a consultation with your healthcare provider for a medical perspective, and provide reputable sources for them to explore independently.

Setting clear boundaries about your dietary needs is essential, but communicate these with kindness to avoid misunderstandings. If offered foods outside your diet, politely decline and suggest healthier alternatives. Consistency in these boundaries ensures your loved ones understand and respect your health choices. Involving your friends and family in your health journey can make personal challenges a collective effort. Engage them in your exercise routines or involve them in meal planning and preparation to educate them about nutrition and the benefits of physical activity. Planning a weekly menu together or setting shared health goals like a weekly walk can strengthen your bond and provide mutual motivation.

Enhance their understanding and support by providing educational resources, such as a list of helpful books, websites, and articles. Organizations like the American Diabetes Association offer you and your loved ones valuable information. Sharing success stories of others who have managed diabetes well can also be inspiring. By involving your friends and family in your lifestyle changes and equipping them with knowledge, you transform their support into a powerful tool for maintaining health improvements, creating a supportive environment that fosters long-term health and wellness.

8.4 ADJUSTING YOUR PLAN AS YOU AGE

Tailoring Your Health Plan as You Age

As we age, our bodies experience significant changes that influence our metabolism, physical capabilities, and nutritional needs. These alterations necessitate a strategic approach to managing blood sugar and weight. With metabolism slowing down over the years, adjusting caloric intake and physical activity becomes crucial to prevent unwanted weight gain and spikes in blood sugar levels. Modifying your diet to suit a slower metabolism might include reducing portion sizes or limiting high-calorie foods.

Additionally, aging can alter how your body processes food, often leading to a heightened carbohydrate sensitivity. It's advisable to monitor your carb intake closely, opting for foods with a lower glycemic index to keep blood sugar levels stable. Increasing your fiber intake can also mitigate the impact of these metabolic changes by slowing sugar absorption into your bloodstream.

Maintaining an active lifestyle is essential, though the nature of your exercise regimen may need to evolve. High-impact activities may become less suitable, making it important to find alternatives that support mobility, strength, and cardiovascular health without straining the joints. Low-impact exercises such as swimming, cycling, resistance band workouts, and yoga are beneficial for managing weight and blood sugar and enhancing overall mobility and quality of life.

Strength training becomes increasingly vital as you age to offset muscle mass loss, which can commence in your 30s and accelerate with time. Muscle tissue is more metabolically active than fat, helping to maintain a healthy weight and metabolic rate. Incorporate weight-bearing and resistance exercises into your weekly routine to support muscle mass. Activities like using weights, bodyweight exercises, or even gardening and light shoveling can be effective forms of resistance training.

Ensuring Bone and Muscle Health Advancing age also raises the concern of osteoporosis and diminishing bone density, especially in post-menopausal women, though it's a universal issue. Adequate calcium and vitamin D intake is key for bone health, and it is achievable through dairy, green leafy vegetables, fortified foods, and sensible sun exposure. Depending on your health and diet, supplements may be necessary, but consult a healthcare provider before starting.

Regular physical activity, particularly weight-bearing exercises, strengthens bones and muscles, maintains metabolic health, and improves balance. This can help reduce the risk of falls and injuries, which become more concerning as we age. Adjusting your health management plan over time is about both responding to and preparing for the natural changes in your body. You can maintain vitality, stable blood sugar, and a robust body by adapting your diet and exercise routines and monitoring health indicators. This proactive strategy ensures your health plan evolves with you, supporting your well-being at every stage of life.

8.5 THE IMPORTANCE OF CONTINUOUS LEARNING AND ADAPTATION

In an ever-evolving landscape of health and science, staying updated on the latest research in diabetes and metabolic health is essential. This continuous learning isn't just about absorbing new information; it's about actively applying it to enhance and potentially simplify health management. Discoveries in dietary strategies or innovative exercises could significantly impact blood sugar stabilization and weight loss efforts.

Navigating the influx of new information requires discernment and prioritizing evidence-based sources such as medical journals, trusted health news sites, and professional recommendations. Engaging with diabetes education newsletters and attending relevant workshops and seminars can also offer valuable, actionable insights.

Incorporating new strategies or technologies into your health plan demands critical evaluation to ensure alignment with your health goals and status. For example, a new fitness tracker providing detailed activity and blood sugar level insights could be beneficial if its efficacy and safety are confirmed. Consultation with healthcare providers is crucial to make informed decisions on integrating new methods into your health regimen.

Adaptation is key in managing diabetes and metabolic health. It requires flexibility to new information, technologies, and personal health changes. This adaptive mindset views changes as opportunities for improvement, encouraging experimentation with new approaches while closely monitoring their health impact.

A wealth of resources for deepening understanding of diabetes care is available, from the American Diabetes Association's comprehensive guides to in-depth articles in the "Diabetes Care" journal. Local workshops, seminars, online forums, and social media groups provide community support and a platform for sharing experiences.

These resources keep you informed and connected to a supportive community, reinforcing motivation and enabling you to maintain healthy gains for a vibrant, active lifestyle.

8.6 CELEBRATING YOUR SUCCESS AND PLANNING FOR THE FUTURE

In life's journey, each health victory, regardless of size, is a crucial milestone worth celebrating. Acknowledging achievements like improved A1C levels, weight loss, or consistent diet management boosts your determination to persist. Simple rewards, such as a new book or a nature outing, reinforce the value of your efforts.

Setting new goals in alignment with these victories keeps your progress in motion. For example, weight training or yoga could enhance blood sugar control and overall strength. Exploring diabetic-friendly recipes or learning about portion control can also be beneficial. These goals prevent regression and encourage continuous improvement.

It's essential to envision your long-term health goals, a future with vibrant activity levels, minimal health issues, or the ability to enjoy time with your family. Outline practical steps to achieve this vision, focusing on cardiovascular health, weight management, and blood glucose control. This foresight motivates daily choices and keeps you on track.

Sharing your journey with others through personal conversations, blogs, or social media amplifies your success and motivates your circle. Your experience could inspire someone to embark on or persist in their health journey, fostering a wellness community.

This cycle of achieving, celebrating, and setting new goals ensures the sustainability of your health improvements. Each step forward builds on the last, guiding you towards a healthier, more fulfilled life. Remember, your journey enhances your well-being and inspires those around you, creating a ripple effect of health and happiness.

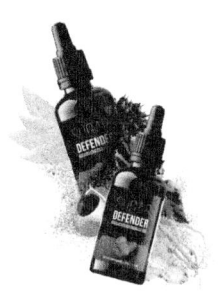

Please click the link and visit the website if you need more information. You can also order the products only from the website.

Click the link or copy and paste it into your browser.

https://hop.clickbank.net/?affiliate=hentom56&vendor=sugardef&pid=pre1

Your Experience Matters!

You're firmly on the pathway to better health and happiness, and that puts you in the perfect position to inspire others to find it too.

Simply by sharing your honest opinion of this book and a little about your own experience, you'll let other readers know just how possible transformation really is, and you'll inspire them to take the first steps on their own journey.

IN UNDER 1 MINUTE
YOU CAN HELP OTHERS JUST LIKE YOU BY LEAVING A REVIEW!

Thank you so much for your support. I wish you a lifetime of good health and happiness.

Scan the QR code or follow this link to leave a review:

https://www.amazon.com/review/create-review/?asin=B0DBD3RGS1

Conclusion

As we draw this guide to a close, I want to take a moment to reflect on the transformative journey you've embarked upon. From unraveling the complexities of blood sugar and its profound impact on body weight to adopting a holistic lifestyle that champions dietary changes, physical activity, and mental well-being, you've taken significant strides toward a healthier you. This journey is not just about understanding science; it's about integrating that knowledge into a vibrant and sustainable life.

Throughout this book, we've explored critical aspects of managing blood sugar and facilitating weight loss. We delved into the importance of a balanced, low-GI diet, consistent physical activity, and the benefits of quality sleep and effective stress management. Each of these elements doesn't just contribute to better blood sugar control; they weave together to form a holistic approach to health that supports every part of your being.

A key component of your journey has been the introduction of Sugar Defender, a natural ally in your quest for health. Remember, incorporating Sugar Defender into your daily routine supports achieving and maintaining your blood sugar and weight management goals. Its natural formulation complements the changes you're making, providing a foundation that helps stabilize blood sugar levels naturally.

However, the path to optimal health doesn't end here. Staying abreast of the latest research in blood sugar management and being willing to adapt your strategies are crucial as you move forward. The landscape of health and wellness is continually evolving, and so should our approaches to managing our well-being.

Maintaining the changes you've made requires consistent effort. It's important to view this not as a temporary diet or a passing phase but as a permanent shift towards a healthier lifestyle. The journey to better health is ongoing; consistency is your greatest ally in achieving long-term success. I encourage you to integrate the knowledge and strategies from this book into your daily life. Share your journey with others, inspire those around you, and build a community of support and encouragement. Your story can motivate others to make similar positive changes, creating ripples extending far beyond your life.

I invite you to share your feedback on this book and your personal stories of transformation. Your experiences not only enrich your life but also help others who are on similar paths. For additional resources, support groups, or online communities focused on blood sugar management and natural health weight loss, continue to explore and engage with platforms that offer support and information.

In closing, I sincerely thank you for trusting this book as your guide and for your commitment to taking control of your health. I hope that this book has provided you with valuable insights and practical tools that will support you on your journey to a healthier, more vibrant life. Remember, every step you take is a step towards a better you. With warmest regards and best wishes for your continued health and well-being,

References

- *Study on the Correlation between Metabolism, Insulin ...* https://www.ncbi.nlm.nih.gov/pmc/articles/PMC7674895/
- *10 Supplements to Help Lower Blood Sugar* https://www.healthline.com/nutrition/blood-sugar-supplements
- *Effect of glycemic index on satiety and body weight - SciELO* https://www.scielo.br/j/rn/a/dVXP9KJD7HXqyTRBgJXW7dq/#:~:text=Short%2Dterm%20investigations%20have%20generally,than%20high%20glycemic%20index%20foods.
- *Watch Out! - Sugar Defender Reviews, Risks & Benefits 2024* https://chrodis.eu/sponsored/sugar-defender-reviews-healthy-blood-sugar-pros-cons-ingredients/
- *Low Glycemic Diet: Its Effects, What to Eat and Avoid, and More* https://www.healthline.com/nutrition/low-glycemic-diet
- *Finding the Hidden Sugar in the Foods You Eat* https://www.hopkinsmedicine.org/health/wellness-and-prevention/finding-the-hidden-sugar-in-the-foods-you-eat
- *How Fiber Helps Manage Diabetes* https://www.verywellhealth.com/soluble-and-insoluble-fiber-1087462
- *Dietary fat, insulin sensitivity and the metabolic syndrome* https://pubmed.ncbi.nlm.nih.gov/15297079/
- *Diabetes diet: Create your healthy-eating plan* https://www.mayoclinic.org/diseases-conditions/diabetes/in-depth/diabetes-diet/art-20044295
- *Low-GI recipes* https://www.bbcgoodfood.com/recipes/collection/low-gi-recipes
- *Diabetes Meal Planning & Batch Cooking* https://www.mynmchealth.org/diabetes-meal-planning-batch-cooking/
- *Artificial sweeteners and other sugar substitutes* https://www.mayoclinic.org/healthy-lifestyle/nutrition-and-healthy-eating/in-depth/artificial-sweeteners/art-20046936
- *Understanding Blood Glucose and Exercise | ADA* https://diabetes.org/health-wellness/fitness/blood-glucose-and-exercise

REFERENCES

- *Lack of Sleep and Diabetes - Sleep Foundation* https://www.sleepfoundation.org/physical-health/lack-of-sleep-and-diabetes
- *Managing Stress When You Have Diabetes* https://www.webmd.com/diabetes/managing-stress
- *Evaluation of a novel supplement to reduce blood glucose ...* https://www.ncbi.nlm.nih.gov/pmc/articles/PMC3056567/
- *10 Supplements to Help Lower Blood Sugar* https://www.healthline.com/nutrition/blood-sugar-supplements
- *What to Know About Sugar and Depression - WebMD* https://www.webmd.com/diet/what-to-know-about-sugar-and-depression
- *Diabetes diet: Create your healthy-eating plan* https://www.mayoclinic.org/diseases-conditions/diabetes/in-depth/diabetes-diet/art-20044295
- *Blood Glucose and Exercise - American Diabetes Association* https://diabetes.org/health-wellness/fitness/blood-glucose-and-exercise
- *14 Easy Ways to Lower Blood Sugar Levels Naturally* https://www.healthline.com/nutrition/14-ways-to-lower-blood-sugar
- *undefined* undefined
- *Changing a Community: A Holistic View of the ...* https://www.ncbi.nlm.nih.gov/pmc/articles/PMC10449002/
- *Understanding Blood Glucose and Exercise | ADA* https://diabetes.org/health-wellness/fitness/blood-glucose-and-exercise
- *Intermittent fasting for weight loss in people with type 2 diabetes* https://www.nih.gov/news-events/nih-research-matters/intermittent-fasting-weight-loss-people-type-2-diabetes
- *Effects of the Ketogenic Diet on Glycemic Control in ...* https://www.ncbi.nlm.nih.gov/pmc/articles/PMC7641470/
- *Understanding Advanced Carbohydrate Counting* https://www.todaysdietitian.com/newarchives/120913p40.shtml
- *The 10 biggest diabetes tech stories from 2023* https://www.drugdeliverybusiness.com/10-biggest-diabetes-tech-stories-2023/
- *10 Supplements to Help Lower Blood Sugar* https://www.healthline.com/nutrition/blood-sugar-supplements
- *Maintenance of lost weight and long-term management ...* https://www.ncbi.nlm.nih.gov/pmc/articles/PMC5764193/
- *Metabolism Changes With Age, Just Not When You Might Think* https://today.duke.edu/2021/08/metabolism-changes-age-just-not-when-you-might-think

REFERENCES

- *How to Talk to Your Family About Dietary Restrictions* https://www.ariaintegrative.com/2019/11/24/how-to-talk-to-your-family-about-dietary-restrictions/
- Page, Seraine. "57 Quotes on Wellness and Health to Inspire Healthy Living." Total Wellness. Last modified January 13, 2022. https://info.totalwellnesshealth.com/blog/quotes-on-wellness-and-health

Printed in Great Britain
by Amazon